EVE JUNIPER

A Practical Guide for Women to Start Practicing Yoga after 40

The Simple, Empowering Path to More Ease, Strength & Confidence From The First Time You Step Onto Your Mat

First edition

This book was professionally typeset on Reedsy.
Find out more at reedsy.com

*To all the strong women on their path to
re-connecting with their Higher Selves.*

*And to my sister and best friend Sandra.
Thank you for introducing me to the art of Yoga 15 years ago.
You continue to inspire me with your strength, your patience and grace,
and the bright light within you.
I love you so much.*

Remember, it doesn't matter how deep into a posture you go — what does matter is who you are when you get there.

MAX STROM

Contents

1

MY GIFT TO YOU

YOGA
MOVEMENT &
MEDITATION

nourish body, mind & soul

To get you started on your Yoga mat and put into practice what you're learning in this book, I would love to invite you to join me online. At the end of the book, you'll find how access your free gift.

I look forward to seeing you on the inside!

2

INTRODUCTION

Welcome to my practical guide for every woman after 40 who would like to start a Yoga practice but is unsure or fearful or lack the confidence to believe she can do this. Many women have been where you are now, including myself, and have found incredible results from a consistent Yoga practice. So I'm extremely excited to share this book.

I've always had this huge urge to share *so* much when new students walk through the door, literally everything you'll find in this book. I realise though, there is only so much one can take in, especially in that first class:

- I'm excited for you to be here, for taking the step to show up for yourself. Whatever it was that brought you here.
- I want to empower you. You *can* absolutely do this.
- I share with you ways to get curious about yourself, and your intelligent and truly fascinating body and mind.
- I want to help you get back control over the endless loop of limiting thoughts, worries and concerns in your mind.

- I will shed light on many aspects of the practice so you can deepen and improve your practice from the first time you step onto your mat.

I get so excited as I know how life-changing the practice can be – as it has been for me over and over again. So now I have the perfect pocket-sized book to give to all my new students, so I can share all the things I would LOVE to share with you in that first class. I'll probably print out some copies and make them available for you when you join my class.

The second reason why I'm so excited to write this book is that it is the trialed and tested foundation of what I have taught and seen amazing results with over the past 15 years of teaching and practicing Yoga and Meditation. It almost feels like universal truth to me and I keep coming back to it over and over. In my teachings as well as in my own practice.

It aims to serve as a great starting point to dive deep into your own experiences. Physically and mentally. It will **not** teach you any postures – this I will do online or in person - your invitation awaits at the end of the book!

It's a guide to shift perception, even before you step onto your mat. To get started today. For a variety of practical situations on and off the mat, it will help you gain confidence, find ease and joy in the process as well as trust in yourself. I'll be the little voice in the back of your mind that encourages you to keep going, to stay and become more curious, and to never give up on yourself.

Our bodies and minds change as we move through our thirties and forties. So does our focus, our intentions, our perceptions, and often our whole outlook on life.

3

This book is not a book on Peri or Menopause. However, as it's been very much a big part of my own journey, I will mention it as Yoga has been a vital tool that helped me navigate this time with more ease and grace.

I was 37 when my world was turned upside down. As you can imagine, I had no idea what was going on at first. Since then, I have learned to welcome it as a kind, friendly guide into the next chapter of my life.

Did you know that Menopause starts around 10 years leading up to the point it actually happens? On average this is around the age of 51. So if you're 40+, it's something that will slowly start to present itself in your life. Sometimes, it happens much earlier. Sometimes you'll notice it, sometimes the symptoms won't express until later on. It is very different for all of us.

The thing is that still to this day, most of us are simply not prepared to move through this big new chapter of our lives - with ease. I have only recently had a dear friend of mine ask me about it - in shock as she had no idea it could come up as early as the late thirties. So what I hear everywhere is that Menopause or Perimenopause are not talked about as much as they should. And oftentimes when it is, the narrative around it is one of "battling it out" or "beating Menopause". Many women experience this time as a nuisance, an unavoidable, unfair act of life. Suffering, in fight and flight mode, being annoyed the inconvenience of it, fighting their bodies, in a state of shock, symptom overload, and misunderstanding as to what is going on.

I would love to invite you to take a different approach: Menopause doesn't have to be beaten or conquered!

Instead, it's an invitation to go on a transformational and empowering journey to get to know yourself on a deeper level, stand tall and walk this new path in your life with strength, grace, openness and a whole lot of self-love. As Marianne Williamson says: You are powerful beyond measure. I second that!

Let's make it part of our conversations, let's be part of the change! Join a group, either in person or online. Seek out classes, women circles, podcasts and books. Ask questions, be curious, talk to your daughters, granddaughters and nieces about it. Lift them up instead of making them "dread the time they cannot avoid".

I hope you'll find a way to embrace it and grow and thrive as a result. There is a powerful wisdom within that time, however challenging it often is. I'll be sure to add some further reading for you in the resource section.

With the help of this practical book and the tips and exercises, as well as the physical practice with me online, I aim to encourage you to open your mind to a way that allows you to walk your path with more ease. Whether you are going through Menopause or not yet. Or you've already come out the other side.

Let's start by creating a foundation for your body and mind for more equanimity in the process. Open yourself up to the possibility of "allowing". Allowing it all to be ok just as it is, and also seeing purpose along the way. Consider it an empowering alternative to "fighting" whatever experience you're going through.

It won't always be easy, though with courage, shifts in perception, and trust, you pave the way for less frustration and suffering along the way.

Be brave lovely one, keep on moving forward. Give yourself permission to welcome it all in.

Allow it all to be part of the experience of being alive. At this and every moment in time.

This book is packed with practical advice for you to dive in to start your physical Yoga practice as a beginner. A ton of information eagerly awaits you to be soaked up. Move ahead and leave behind any expectations you have that might hold you back from getting started right now.

Thank you for your presence. It is an honour to guide you as you embark on this life-changing path.

3

READ, REFLECT AND PRACTICE

And repeat. Take your time, there's no need to rush it. Maybe you feel like reading it in one go, by all means. Take it as a guide to support you with your intentions for your time on the mat.

Even though it's an easy read, you might find that some of the information will only sink in once you unroll your mat and start practicing. That's the idea behind it, though all is good. Simply come back to it again.

Place your book close to your Yoga mat or wherever you'll be practicing. Read a section or chapter, five or ten minutes before you step onto your mat.

There will be good days and bad days. Happy blissful hours. And grey and difficult times with limiting thoughts that want to bring you down. Take a breath. Take note. Reflect. Write down anything that comes up. Get yourself a notebook or diary, especially for your Yoga practice, let it be your ally and witness alongside you on this journey.

In the next chapters, we talk about expanding our awareness of ourselves and creating conscious, mindful moments in our practice and our life too. When you practice with me, you will often hear me say words like: "Notice", "Consider how...", "Observe". They're invitations to reflect, observe and dive into the space you're discovering within you.

Take a deep breath in
Exhale it all out

A deeper awareness is the entry point for a deeper experience of ourselves. Being aware of ourselves is the only way we get to really know ourselves. It means being mindful, being present, open to each experience as it presents itself. And of course, without judgment or analysing - simply loving and accepting who and where we are.

It doesn't have to be more complicated than that. When practicing, you take the time and space to observe, discover and experience yourself. You're creating a powerful relationship with yourself. Don't worry if you're unsure what that looks like right now. There is no right or wrong. Nothing needs to be different than it is. You don't need to be stronger or more flexible or more graceful. The most important thing is for you to notice what is. Connect with that part of yourself and allow it to be there.

Whatever you need to learn and understand, to process and grow, it won't run away, you won't miss it. It will keep coming back to you. However much you think you 'fail', however many mistakes you make, or however long it takes. Don't become disheartened. You will learn in time as your body and mind become stronger and more open to integrate it all.

"When the student is ready, the teacher appears".

This quote is said to be by Lao Tzu's Tao Te Ching. It alludes to the fact that we only take in what we have the capacity to comprehend at any stage in our learning and development. It's the same on the mat. There's no need to take it all in at once.

Along the way, simply reflect on whatever comes up: Any reactions when you don't understand something the teacher says. Notice your mind on good days vs bad days. Notice your mind if and when your body isn't able to go where your mind wants it to. When your neighbour seems to be doing everything so much more graceful than you. What happens in your mind at the time? How do you react?

Train yourself to really listen and become deeply aware to it all. Physical sensations, thoughts, emotions, your inner voice and your intuition too - the whole experience. How can you cultivate a quality of curiosity to whatever arrives whilst practicing? Be aware of what is here. Right now. Remind yourself of this each time you listen in.

A little side note on so called "mistakes". There are no mistakes. Only learning curves and opportunities for growth. Have you ever noticed in hindsight how you've been repeating a certain 'mistake' over and over until you *got it* and were able to move on? You have probably heard this before, but here you go again: Train yourself to re-frame the word 'mistake' as an opportunity to see the lesson from a different angle. With less judgment - more kindness. Let yourself off the hook and know you're ok and exactly in the right place.

To cultivate that ability to look and listen deeply, more each time you practice, give yourself permission to slow things down and let things settle. Without forcing. Without pushing. Without wanting to be "over there" when in fact, you are right here, still happy discovering the "here and now".

Breathe. Tune in and take your time. One step at a time.

Stay inspired!

In the coming weeks and months of your practice, immerse yourself into your practice, learn more about it. At the end of the book, you'll find several resources for you to dive into, as well as of course my invitation and free gift for you to practice with me online.

Hop onto your mat and let's walk this next step of your journey together. I'll guide you through the physical part of your practice, and together with this book, you can make it a holistic learning experience.

Message me to say hello and let me know where you're at in your practice, as well as how you're progressing as you dive deeper into your Yoga practice. I look forward to meeting you!

"At times your practice will resemble a calm mountain lake, at other times more like the wild waves in the middle of a stormy ocean."

Let's weather the storms together.

4

FAQ'S

How long do I need to practice each week?

When starting out with something new, the amount of new information for body and mind can often feel overwhelming. There is so much to learn, figure out and discover. All the feelings, all the emotions, right? It's exciting, however, it can also very easily result in a massive dose of overwhelm. I'm sure we've all been there. Don't lose motivation! The key is to make it sustainable.

A very easy way to avoid the overwhelm, and also to eradicate any excuses along the way, is to schedule shorter practice times more often. It makes more sense to schedule three 15-minute sessions every week, than three hours once a month.

Create the discipline to make your practice part of your weekly routine. Get excited about it, immerse yourself and remind yourself often of the reason why you practice. You might even find that once you have created a sustainable routine, you might naturally feel the urge to extend your practice time.

Take Action Now !

1. Mark your diary to schedule three 15-minute practices, each week for the next 3 weeks.
2. More if it's sustainable. Any number of times that you can definitely commit to practicing each week. Ideally, make it the same day, same time each week.

Remember that consistency and taking continued action are key when learning anything new and creating new habits.

Where's the best space to practice?

Just as important as *how often* you practice is the *where* you practice. I suggest you practice in the **same space every time**, this could be:

- Anywhere comfortable and safe in your home: your lounge, bedroom or a spare room
- In nature (great for a dose of 'earthing'), maybe your local park or outside in your garden
- When travelling in your hotel room

Be mindful of the surroundings. Make it a place where you're less likely to bump into any objects, chairs, tables or anything that you could possibly hurt yourself on.

If possible, though I realise it's not always that easy with partners, little ones or furry friends running around – **practice somewhere undisturbed.**

Leave your mat rolled out as a loving reminder to practice daily. As you step onto your mat each time - close the door and leave the external world behind.

Take Action Now!

1. Create a designated, undisturbed, cosy and inviting Yoga practice space.
   Have fun with it!
2. Add a blanket and pillow. Even some essential oils and a candle if that's your cup of tea. Oh yes, a cup of tea too.
3. Create a magical, safe space that radiates peace and quality me-time.

A space you love coming back to.

At The Yoga Studio

If you live in town, there will most likely be a wider variety of Yoga Studios and classes in other venues such as church halls, community centres. In the countryside, there's naturally less choice, so to suit a wider audience, a lot of classes are often general and geared for all levels - beginners as well as intermediate and advanced students.

There are a lot of different types of Yoga classes:

- If you see it advertised as Yoga, Hatha or Vinyasa, Gentle, Slow, Iyengar, etc. they're often suitable for beginners. Most will then mention "suitable for beginners" or similar - a great one to start!
- Ashtanga, Forest, Power Yoga, even Hot Yoga, etc all tend to offer a stronger physical practice, yet still suitable for beginners.

If there are no details in the class description, simply call up or email beforehand to check.

And then there are the more specific classes that do what they say on the tin - offering classes for the advertised audience:

- Pregnancy Yoga
- Yoga for Runners (or cyclists or swimmers, … or any other sport)
- Mum & Baby Yoga
- Restorative Yoga (so delicious – do must-try if you're in need of some quality TLC)
- etc.

There are so many other types out there. Don't get discouraged if you tried one class and it didn't quite feel right. It could be for many reasons!

- Maybe it was too big of a challenge.
- Maybe you felt it wasn't challenging enough.
- Maybe you didn't quite gel with the teacher. Trust your intuition! If you have the choice, try another teacher who resonates with you and who might offer what you need at the time.

If you don't have a big choice of which class you can join, I suggest sticking with it! Attend a few sessions and give the teacher a chance. Give yourself a chance! Your perception could change when you start to notice the benefits for your body and mind after a few classes. Put all judgment aside and come with an "attitude of gratitude" towards the teacher. You might be surprised.

What do I wear?

Comfortable clothing

Don't overthink this one. Wear something that makes you feel deliciously good, beautiful and strong. "Stretchy" and not restrictive. You want to be able to move easily, without your clothing holding you back.

Always practice without shoes

The idea is to feel your feet. To feel the connection between yourself and the ground underneath. Practicing without shoes – and without socks - helps to strengthen your proprioception, that sense of where your body is situated in space. You'll improve your balance and generally create a steadier and stronger pose throughout.

There's also a mindful, safety aspect to it. Practicing without socks will help you not to slip on your mat.

Having said all that, not all Yoga studios or community halls are toasty warm. As much as it's fine to go barefoot throughout class when you're warmed up, once you stop moving at the end during Meditation and relaxation, it can feel cold quickly again. If you're anything like me and your feet tend to get cold quickly, put your socks back on (and any other layers you've got if needed).

Please, do not worry if you're the only one (or first one) putting them back on! You might just allow someone to do the same. They will thank you, lovely soul.

Take Action Now!

1. Choose one favourite set of comfy clothes that you feel really good in.
2. Put them all together in one space, so you can quickly get to them without thinking, so they're handy when you're ready to practice.

Do I need a Yoga mat?

Did you know that the Yoga studio industry isworthover $88 billion worldwide?! It's expected to reach $215bn by 2025. If you were to also account for retreats, clothing, mats, blocks, and other props and perks, the global yoga market is worth well over $130bn!

As a result, there is a huge amount of different mats to choose from. You'll find all price ranges, anything your heart desires.

Even though I've always had one or more myself, I've never been very attached to my Yoga mats. Most Yoga studios offer mats for you to use. So if you're on a tight budget, don't worry as you don't necessarily need one right now.

The main thing is to make sure you practice on a non-slippery surface. If you can practice outside, on the grass, in nature, connected to the earth – that's my preferred and recommended option. If you've heard of "grounding" or "earthing" before, you will know of the huge effects it has on our health. Do check it out! Of course, practicing outside isn't an option throughout all seasons in a lot of countries.

When practicing inside, practice on a carpet or rug. Again, be mindful of how slippery the surface is. Your experience will be different if you're constantly needing to focus on your feet not sliding away.

You want to be able to create a certain resistance to the ground to increase proprioception, as well as improve awareness of the kinetic chain: Actively root down from your deep inner core through the legs and feet.

In that sense, I would probably encourage you to invest in a Yoga mat. It does make a difference, and because you're on this journey of discovering a new depth to the landscape within you, it'll be a good investment to make.

Discover what works for you.

A short sidenote to *new* Yoga mats: Some mats can start off by actually being a little slippery. Research it before you purchase your own, though don't be concerned or worried or frustrated if you feel you're slipping and sliding extensively when you first start using it. It takes a few weeks to wear it in. Your mat will soon become a good, steady friend to hold and support you.

If you're unsure whether the studio or individual teacher offers mats or not, just get in touch prior to double check. I personally like to bring my own mat, a small towel or a travel mat and a lot of students do the same. This also minimises the question about hygiene.

You'll find that almost all studios provide some sort of disinfectant spray (tea tree is a favourite natural one) to wipe your mat down after class. Just spray it directly onto the mat from a little distance and wipe it. Done. If you are unsure, ask one of the other students, or if you feel too shy, simply hang around an extra moment to see what the others are doing. All good.

What are Yoga 'props'?

Many teachers encourage you to use them and I love them. Some props that you will find in most studios are mats, blocks, straps, bolsters, eye pillows, blankets, knee pads, or wedges.

They act as an extension of the limbs and help you achieve and maintain a healthy structural alignment. And as such they enable you to reap the many benefits of Yoga postures, before your body is willing and strong enough to move deeper. So valuable, not just for beginners, and the kindest and most helpful friends to work with.

The use of them is endless - it's a fun, enriching and valuable experience and I invite you to use them where you can.

Never see them as a 'demotion'. Don't ever think you're not 'good enough' when a teacher suggests using one. Drop the wandering ego mind and notice the difference.

What does it even mean? Common Yoga words and phrases.

Yoga means 'to yoke' or unite. To make whole. It's a spiritual discipline, rather than just moving through a sequence of exercises.

You'll notice that a lot of Yoga terminology is in the Sanskrit language, from ancient yoga texts such as the Yoga Sutras compiled by the sage(s) Patanjali in 2nd / 3rd BCE. There are 196 Sutras, or "threads" which act as a guide or manual that leads toward progressing along ones spiritual path, discovering the true meaning of Yoga, and eventually liberation or enlightenment.

As follows, I very briefly outline a short number of words phrases that you'll probably hear a lot in a Yoga class:

- **Asana:** "Seat". Physical posture or Yoga pose, and the third limb of Patanjali's eightfold path (Ashtanga)
- **Prana:** Life force or breath.
- **Pranayama:** "life/breath extension". Breath control, or "un-obstructing the breath". The fourth limb of Patanjali's eightfold path
- **Downward dog (Adho Mukha Svanasana):** One of the most common yoga poses. You're on your hands and feet, hips up in an inverted 'V' shape.
- **Surya Namaskar:** "Sun salutations". A beautiful sequence of Yoga postures and probably the most well-known sequences of the Yoga practice. It can be practiced slow and meditative, or as a fast and dynamic warm up and heat building practice.
- **Vinyasa:** 1) it can simply mean "movement linked with breath". 2) It is also described as a certain dynamic sequence within the Sun

Salutation: Chaturanga - Cobra / Upward Facing Dog - Downward Facing Dog. 3) It also describes creative dynamic 'flow' Yoga (not necessarily attached to a particular lineage)

- **Hatha:** "Ha" represents the sun and "tha" represents the moon. It is a branch of Yoga focusing on postures (asana) and breath control (pranayama). As there are little or no flow elements involved, Hatha Yoga tends to be less dynamic and involves holding postures for longer than in a Vinyasa class.

- **Shavasana:** "Corpse pose". Relaxation pose at the end of a Yoga class. (I personally love starting class in Shavasana - a perfect place to check in to see where we're at.)

- **Namaste:** a greeting. One of my favourite translations is: "The divine light within me bows to the divine light within you". Often said as a sign of heartfelt acknowledgment and gratitude at the end of class: bring your palms together in front of your heart, bowing down toward yourself, the teacher and your fellow students.

- **Ujjayi:** "Victorious breath" or "Oceanic breath". Also: "Darth Vada breath" due to the sound it creates as you ever so slightly constrict the back of your throat, breathing in and out through the nose.

- **Chakra:** "Wheel". Energy centres in the body. Yoga is intended to free up the movement of 'prana', our life force, in the body.

- **Mantra:** a word, or sound (for example om) or phrase which can be repeated, a great tool to anchor your mind in meditation

- **Om:** a primordial mantra, sound of the universe, or "universal sound of consciousness". It's the most elemental of vibrations (Gaia) meant to carry immense pranic life force. Often used as 'sound work' and chanted at the beginning and end of yoga classes.

- **Drishti:** gaze or focal point. Used during meditation as well as within the asana practice.

- **Ananda:** a state of utter joy or bliss (experience pockets of that in Shavasana)

5

A BEGINNING. A MIDDLE. AN END.

L ike any good story and pretty much everything else in life, Yoga classes are also structured this way: It's got a beginning, a middle and and an end.

You can pretty much tell from the Yoga poses, whether they're dynamic, static, fast or slow, where you are in your session. Of course it makes sense that our bodies (and minds) are warmed up before jumping into a strong, challenging flow. Also, our Nervous System would be over-stimulated if we were to end the class without taking a moment to rest and process the class and enjoy the space and feelings we're creating during the class. The practice just wouldn't be sustainable or offer the results and benefits it does.

Yoga classes that belong to a certain lineage often have their own, fixed sequences which you'll become familiar with. They will be adjusted according to how long the class is. Though they still follow roughly the same pattern.

Here's a thumb rule how a lot of classes are sequenced:

- **Check In:** Slow down the mind with breathing exercises, disengage from previous activity and bring awareness to the hear and now. Also great to let the body catch up with the mind!
- **Warm Up:** a slow and mindful sequence of postures to warm up muscles and joints to prepare the body for the physical practice - according to the theme or focus of each class.
- **Flow element:** A more dynamic flow to generate heat in the body (can also be achieved with certain breathing exercises). Often, these are any variation of the Sun Salutations.
- **Flow:** In a Vinyasa class, this can be a creative flow, movements connected to the breath, to build up to a certain pose that's being practiced, or to express the theme of the class. It's generally more 'yang' then 'yin'
- **Static or Yin poses, cool down:** slow down holding the poses for longer, work on flexibility, breathe and allow opening to happen. As you can imagine, this one is more 'yin' then 'yang'
- **Relaxation or Shavasana:** Put any layers back on if you get cold easily before you get into this last pose of the class: 'Corpse Pose'. Not the most inviting name, however, it explains well what you're doing: Lie on your back, supported with pillows and blankets. The teacher might guide you through a last body scan to help relax all parts of the body. Notice for another moment the buzzing throughout your body, the space, the ease, the feeling of accomplishment of the practice you've just completed and the wonderful feeling you created within. Now there's nothing else to do, simply drop in and enjoy the silence for a while longer. (Side note: often utter bliss).

For a moment here, let's peak our head out beyond the Yoga class setting into our lives. We're not often as conscious about our activities. We mindlessly jump from one activity to the next, filling our days with work and endless to-do lists, accompanied by a sea of distractions, and then at the end of a busy week we feel guilty for not getting it all done. Without ever stopping and consciously arriving, we're running the risk of missing the sweetest and most important moments and opportunities in our lives.

So here's my invitation for you:

For your new adventure on the mat, I invite you to actively consider and cultivate awareness of the beginning (and the "before"), the middle ("during") and the end ("closing") of your practice. Be present, be here now. Show up for yourself fully. Don't just go through the motions. Keep coming back to your breath. Don't judge yourself if your mind wanders, instead keep coming back home to yourself.

As you continue reading, take one aspect at a time to focus on throughout your practice on the mat. Notice what comes up, journal it, notice how things change over time. But most of all, notice what happens from taking disciplined and focused action. You're setting the ball rolling and soon the immense benefits of the practice will start flowing in.

Through your physical practice, you *will* start to reap the more well-known benefits like becoming more flexible and mobile, stronger and more resilient. From the very first time onward. Whether that's very noticeable to you to begin with or not, it is happening. With a consistent practice, you are beginning to cultivate change on a deeper level. On an physical as well as an energetic level.

Don't rush ahead

Enjoy discovering your inner landscape and take time to let your experience settle and grow. Whilst practicing be present for the tough and intense times too. Whether these are of physical or mental or emotional nature. They're all part of the experience of what makes your life a rich and well-lived one.

Breathe. Stand tall. I've got your back. Let's get started.

The Beginning - Before You Practice

One of the aspects of our Yoga practice is to cultivate awareness. Creating and deepening it starts with knowing (i.e., being aware of) where you are right now.

Here's an easy tool to cultivate awareness, something I encourage you to do often. Make it a habit, each time you step onto your mat.

Check-in With Yourself

Do it with me right now:

Take a moment to stop.
   Disengage from any previous activities.
   Take a few deep breaths. In through the nose. Out through the mouth.
   Inhale deeply. Exhale let go.
   Notice anything that comes up. Any sensations.
   Within your body. Your breath.
   Notice how you feel temperature-wise. Your energy.
   How active is your mind right now?
   Scan your body from the crown of your head down to the feet.

Slow it down.
Cultivate a sense of curiosity for your inner happenings.

Check-in often.

Your breath will help you to move into parasympathetic nervous system mode. You'll more easily create focus and clarity as well as a feeling of being more centred and grounded.

You'll soon notice how checking in with yourself will help you become aware of the areas within you that most need your attention at this moment. You'll *know* what exactly it is that you need today.

The more you practice checking in, the deeper your awareness becomes. The quicker you notice anything that feels off, the quicker you can do something about it before it turns into a niggle, an injury, or even an illness.

Intention

A wonderful tool to add to every session is creating an intention for your practice. Sometimes the teacher will suggest one at the beginning of class. Though even if they don't, it's a powerful habit to cultivate.

Here's how!

Think of a quality or a feeling you would like to cultivate in your life. Take a moment to tune in and become conscious of what it is you want to create. In your body. Your mind. Your whole life.

It could simply be that you would like to send some love and energy to a loved one, someone who could benefit from it right now.

Sankalpa is a concept in Yoga Philosophy that refers to an intention formed by the heart and mind. It starts with the radical premise that you are enough already. You already are perfect. You already are who you need to be to fulfill your life's work or your purpose in life.

When setting an intention, give it a positive spin. Look for qualities you'd like to amplify in your life. Word them in a way as if they have already happened. As if they're already a part of your life. You might not have the experience in your physical life just yet, but imagine you do! State it in present tense. Really *feel* into it and imagine how it makes you feel having these *be* your reality right now.

Remind yourself of your intention throughout your practice. Breathe in its essence, soak it up, allow it to swallow you whole and then embody it fully. Let it carry you through your whole practice.

"I move with intention"

The Middle - During Your Practice

The below aspects are a selection of the top nuggets of wisdom I love sharing with my students in class. It's by no means complete. Though for now, go ahead and soak them up and come back to them often.

Your Breath

Maintain a strong, conscious breath at all times. Practice long breaths, smooth and even. Like the ebb and flow of a calm ocean.

This single mindful breath is also a powerful meditative tool that acts as a switch from your sympathetic state ('s' for stress) to a more parasympathetic state ('p' for peace). To encourage healing on all levels. Continuously notice when the quality of your breath changes:

- Are you holding your breath or are you breathing very shallowly?
- Does it feel choppy, uneven or laboured?

If it does, back up a bit and ask yourself:

- How can I be here and still breathe long, smooth, even breaths?
- How can I allow myself to be here, without the running commentary of my mind? What can I focus on instead?

If you need to, take a short break to re-connect. Don't be shy, even when you're in a studio class. **Make your breath the single most important priority throughout your practice.**

Sensations as Tools for Deeper Awareness

Any sensations within our body are a welcomed opportunity for reflection.

I still remember showing up to my first class in a village hall in the south of England, feeling really clumsy, unflexible and oh so uncomfortable. I looked around, men and women of all ages, all of whom clearly seemed to know what they were doing. All of them looked so graceful compared to my awkward self. It felt weird at the time, I was fit and in good shape from a lot of running, I even used to do gymnastics when I was younger. Surely that must count for something…? Why did I feel so out of place?? How can I make it to the end of this class without making a fool of myself?? My mind was racing and I was wondering how to get into all the different shapes and forms, whilst my body gave me the unmistakable signal that it just didn't want to. Nope. I felt weak, trembling in the easiest-looking exercises! Argh, how could it all be so difficult?!

All the feelings. All the emotions. It was intense. I remember it very clearly.

Focusing outward might be the initial reaction, looking at what other students do or compare yourself to them. In the past 12+ years of teaching, I've come to see many in the same boat. For your first class, see how you can stay with yourself, your own physical sensations. Soften the grip of your mind. Drop all expectations and leave your inner judge outside.

Whenever you notice your mind wandering or that critical pesky inner voice appears that tries to put you down, bring it back to focus on your own movements, your own body, and your breath. Take it easy, one breath at a time.

Know that all the physical sensations that arise within are key parts of the puzzle that is *you*. Simply notice. Also how they change and shift within class as well as over time. Maybe your thinking mind joins you with a running commentary on everything. Maybe you'll even have some of my own thoughts and experience come up for you.

And if you do, wrap yourself into a blanket of love and kindness, and tell yourself it's all good. Remind yourself to not take yourself too seriously. Smile and see the fun side of it. After all, you're an explorer now courageously navigating the edge of your comfort zone! A little lightness will make journey a lot easier.

Body Scan

A body scan are a powerful type of meditation that help us dive in to noticing on a deeper level any sensations or feelings as they arise in the body. It's as simple as scanning your body from head to toe. They are a regular part of a Yoga practice and the teacher will often lead you through such a meditation towards the end, before Shavasana, to relax fully. The focus on the physical body acts as an anchor for the mind, encouraging peace and relaxation throughout. As such they are a wonderful practice if you have trouble falling or staying asleep at night.

Tune in and follow the journey to *feel* into your body. From the top of your head, down to the feet. And up again. Feel anything that comes up. Anything that's most dominant. Anything that comes and goes. Anything that lingers for a while. Maybe even any intense or even painful sensations. Try not to fidget or give into the urge to adjust if you don't need to.

Get curious and for a moment, try to express in words what exactly the sensations feel like. Maybe you can pinpoint them in your mind's eye, seeing where exactly they are or where they come from. With as little judgment as possible, take every moment as it comes.

The more often you practice scanning the body, the more familiar you'll get with your own sensations, and the better you get to know yourself.

The body scan will get easier within the postures as well as throughout the movements during your practice. Over time, it will become second nature to scan the body often and instantly. You'll start to develop a curious *knowing*, an energetic sense of all the sensations at once. You'll know instantly how to adjust, you'll know with the slightest 'off' feeling what to do to move towards balance again. You're slowly starting to discover this powerful guidance system within you.

For now, keep checking in with yourself throughout your practice. There's no need to race through a whole body scan every time. Simply linger in one place for a while and notice any shifts along the way, however minute they are. And then move ahead with your practice.

I have created several beautiful Guided Meditations to really practice this art of tuning in. Follow the link in the resource section for how to access them.

Your Powerful Guidance System

Within your practice on the mat, you're moving through a variety of movements, some of which can be very deep, to open your body up and start generating power from a deeper place, from the inner body within. And the deeper you can generate power from, the more strength, ease, and awareness you can create in your outer body.

As you continue tuning in, you'll start to detect this powerful guidance system I mentioned earlier. It'll allow you to trust yourself more, increase your intuition and really deepen the relationship with yourself. And over time, this will reveal a huge inner wisdom you can always rely on.

As you can imagine, there are a lot of subtleties when it comes to the signals and sensations that our body sends us all the time. Warm delicious feel-good feelings of ease and grace. Or: discomfort, niggles, aches, and of course pain too!

The latter feelings are the signals that arise when we move toward the edge of our comfort zone. Our comfort zone is that cosy place where we feel safe and secure. Imagine it as a bubble within the *great, scary unknown*.

The question is, of course, whether to stay inside cosy-comfy? Or to venture out? Be brave, beautiful soul, venture out and see what's out there!

The Edge

During your practice, we're being challenged to find this edge. Every single time. Whether it's strength, or flexibility, whether that's in your body or your mind.

Yes, sometimes it's a scary place to hang out. It's got a tendency to relentlessly bring you face to face with your insecurities, feelings of vulnerability, weakness, and fear. You might feel the strong pull to turn around and get back into your comfort zone, the known, feeling safe again.

Can you stay here for a while?
Lean into it and embrace it

Play with your edge and lighten up. There's good news! Our edge is also the place you get to grow!

As you tickle the edge, whether you just look across it or jump in head first - notice the freedom, the liberation that comes with it. The strength you develop. Instantly. The ease with which you can breathe easier and deeper. You're creating space and lightness in your body. You're learning to soften into the struggle and resistance, maybe even leaving it behind completely along the way.

The longer you hang out there, the easier it will be to open up to the potential and opportunities and the life that awaits you on the other side. Physically as well as mentally and emotionally.

Imagine the following scenario:

You're on your yoga mat and realise that as easy as this position looks, it's actually really hard to get into. Even worse, once you manage to catapult yourself into it somehow – it's really tough to hold for as long as the teacher suggests. Your breath is heavy, you feel totally out of sync. You feel physically stuck, as you attempt to let it vaguely resemble what, gauged from the corners of your eyes, seemingly all other students in class manage to gracefully and effortlessly achieve.

We've all been there when we first started. And that's wonderful! Remember how it feels!

My invitation to you is to not go into freak-out mode. Let go of any expectations and just come as you are. Step into the challenge. Embrace it. With all of your strengths and with all of your weaknesses. Leave self-doubt at the door, as well as all self-limiting, judgmental, and all other negative thoughts and vibes. Acknowledge them, tell them good bye and then bring your focus back.

The magic lies in **creating a strong foundation** within each pose and then finding a way how to hang out there, within the intensity of your edge. Breathe, lovely one. Remember, here's exactly where you grow. If it's way too much, if you've gone way over your edge, back up a bit. Work on expanding your comfort zone, establishing your foundation at the edge and soon your body will be willing and able to progress further.

Our Yoga practice is so much about creating graceful resilience and equanimity - ease of mind. Standing strong during the storm, feeling the intensity of each pose.

Be gentle with yourself. Stay just a little longer. You can do it.

And maybe along the lines, you can start to consider: Can I enjoy these moments? Even the challenging ones? How can I celebrate them for being an exquisite part of my experience at this very moment?

Let's take Plank Pose, for example, a challenging core and whole-body strength pose. If you're not used to holding it, your body might react by shaking like a leaf.

It is right at that point where you know you're close to your edge. Don't freak out, but again – can you observe what's happening? Start to find a gentle gaze forward ('drishti') and breathe. Long, controlled, strong inhalations and exhalations. Stay with your breath. Scan your body and breathe. Inhale. Exhale. You can do this.

Our edge is the place where not only we get stronger, but we also create discipline and focus. We're changing our muscular design and literally altering the chemistry in our bodies.

It won't be long until you'll get familiar with the basic shapes of the postures and the sequences you'll move through. You will soon be able to consciously connect your breaths and moving with more precision. And along the way you'll gain strength, and find more effortlessness to breathe fully and freely.

Take it easy. As with everything it's practice, practice, practice.

Grateful Pain

There's a whole range of 'pain' sensations and of course, it's a topic in and of itself. Being able to differentiate them will come with time and curiosity, as you continue stepping onto your mat to practice. You'll get better at reading the sensations, signs, and signals as they happen.

There's for example muscular soreness or discomfort that may arise through lack of use or overuse. For example after a big training session or a strong Yoga class for example. It's usually more of a broad, dull feeling, yet can often be very deep.

Of course, there are also many nuances within that, though generally, it's the type of pain that's also called *grateful pain*. It's a result of your body moving into a range that it's not used to anymore, for a little too long, so the next day you might be feeling it.

The grateful pain is the *good kinda pain*. Where you know you've tickled the edge of your comfort zone. Nothing to worry about. Yet you still want to be very mindful of course.

And then there's the type of pain that you do *not* want to come across.

This type of sensation is a bit punchier. It's a sudden, sharp feeling that comes with stepping beyond what your body is happy to do at that point. There's a risk it might turn into a more consistent niggle or even an injury. Or maybe it already has when you feel it. A signal that was ignored, a step pushed too far.

We've got these incredible natural mechanisms within our bodies, that aim toward preventing us from getting hurt or injured (for example by compensating or creating resistance in the body). However, often there's also a strength of the (ego) mind which believes it's ok to ignore this resistance. That part of the mind that thinks it's ok to push and force it a little more.

Please don't. Your Yoga mat isn't 'no pain no gain' territory. Don't push against the resistance. Never force yourself into a stretch. The tightness doesn't need to be "conquered". All you'll do is fight yourself, *against* your body. Creating even more resistance as a result.

If it doesn't feel 'good' (which includes the strong, challenging kind of sensations), don't do it. If it's too much, back up, there might not be a rewind button! Especially if you feel any sharp pain moving in, stop immediately. If you don't know what just happened, check in with your Yoga teacher and it may also be advisable to have it looked at afterwards. Though obviously, this is a situation we want to avoid. We don't want to injure ourselves in a Yoga practice. And it happens more than you think.

So again, instead of pushing deeper or forcing it, ask yourself:

- How can you soften and surrender into the resistance?
- Maybe hang out a little longer to notice how it changes or shifts.
- How can you just be here and breathe for a bit, noticing how any such sensations shift when you do? Do you maybe need to back up even more?

Trust your body. Take your time and listen to work *with* its infinite wisdom and amazingly clever mechanisms. Be patient, and keep breathing. Take back responsibility for your actions and your body. Move with precision and control, give yourself some help along the way, and move mindfully.

When you slowly work your way forward, expanding your comfort zone safely until your body is ready to move on, you'll soon be able to embrace the sensation as such and maybe even start to really enjoy that feeling. The sensations there at the edge won't get less, though you'll know how and who to be there when you come face to face with them. And that's a very empowering place to sit in.

Remember you are creating positive change every time you step onto your mat.

Symmetry & Balance

Every single body is different and comes with its own makeup, its own set of different habits, routines, muscular patterns, and imbalances. Yet there's a certain symmetry in the body that we can all use as a benchmark to work toward more balance and a more natural alignment and with that more power and strength too.

Asymmetry or *imbalance* do not equal wrong or bad. There is no such thing. And if it ain't broke, there's no need to fix it.

However, if it is the cause for pain, discomfort or lack of strength or health in whatever shape it expresses itself, we can choose to slowly move back toward a more optimal posture. And one way to do that is by *countering* the imbalances to bring back balance and harmony.

As always, don't rush it. Take it easy.

It took us our whole lives, no matter how old we are now, to move into this shape and form that we're in now. Through the lifestyles we choose, by sitting at our desks for long hours, hunching forward, and all the circumstances that didn't allow for a more natural posture.

As a result, it will take us a little while to get back to a more optimal form. As I said earlier, be patient. *Know* you're on the right path whilst cultivating a sense of equanimity, a calm and steady mind along the way.

How to Create Balance and Symmetry:

1. Check yourself out and take a visual approach! Scan and notice everything. Maybe you even have a mirror at hand. You will learn how your body moves or reacts in certain situations, postures, or sequences. Wobbly knees, shaking, feeling stuck not getting into (or out of!) a pose, etc.

(A mirror on the other hand might also give fuel to your monkey mind noticing all the things that don't serve you right now. So be mindful of what's most supportive for you here.)

2. As with most things in life, always create a solid foundation first. Be strong. Root down. Then close your eyes whenever it feels safe to do so and dive deep into noticing. How does one side of the body feel compared to the other?

Maybe your left side feels different than the right side? Or vice versa. It's not uncommon at all. And it's not "bad" either. (Don't judge yourself, remember?) It's simply how it presents itself at this moment. It's not a fixed state. And it's one of the very important pieces of the puzzle you're working on creating.

Visualisation

Imagine two little flashlights on both your hip bones, evenly shining forward:

1. Do they continue shining forward when for example you step back into a lunge?
2. How are your hips positioned?
3. Do the flashlights still point forward?
4. Do you need to adjust?
5. Notice the light as you draw one hip forward slightly and the other one back.

Initially, all the cues from your teacher might be a lot to remember.

Don't worry at all – do what you can right now. And work with that first. The rest will come. Next time. And the next. Slowly slowly.

Awareness brings with it a whole world of curious information (aka magic) that you are slowly discovering on your Yoga adventure.

In my classes, I go a little deeper into what balance is and how it can be achieved. For now, simply continue working on creating a deeper awareness of the symmetry and balance in your physical body, without judgment or expectation – notice a sense of intuition, knowing what is right and what feels good for you.

Long Holds

Sometimes, we hold postures a little longer, for a few breaths. You can imagine that the more intense the posture is, the slower time passes. These are "beautiful" times, playing your edge and noticing what arises in your mind!

To start with and to repeat what we talked about earlier - no matter how intense or easy the Yoga pose is - scan your body briefly to check your alignment and foundation. And then, find stillness, by focusing on a smooth, even breath.

Find strength and comfort in the steadiness of your breath. Soften into the intensity of the pose. Be strong.

Relax into areas you don't need right now. As you gain strength and flexibility you will be able to stay (focused) for longer.

Scan. Reflect. Open

1. How do you feel in this moment?
2. Where does your body respond to the structure of the pose?
3. Where do you feel strong?
4. Where do you feel tired?
5. Where are your tight spots?
6. Does one side feel different than the other?
7. What are you learning about yourself?

Transitions

Transitions move us from one Yoga posture to the next. It's easy to discount, though they are just as important as the actual pose, so don't allow your attention to slip moving through them.

Be fully present during every move. Don't rush it.
  Don't catapult yourself forward.
  Don't collapse.
  Don't allow your mind to skip ahead.
  Be here now. Breathe.

Take each moment, each movement as it comes. Move with control – from your core. Breathe and be as meticulous as you can in moving from one pose to the next.

Adjustments & Enhancements

Notice how you feel when being in a pose. Move from side to side a little bit. Play and discover for a little while - what feels natural? What doesn't so much?

Your Yoga teacher will see you and can enhance your practice by giving you pointers and support in deepening the pose. Verbally and hands-on physically.

As good as adjustments often feel, sometimes we'd rather not have anyone move into our space. Here's an important reminder for you:

If you do *not* want the hands-on adjustment from your teacher, for whatever reason, if you feel uncomfortable in any way, be sure to clearly state or signal it to your teacher. A simple "no thank you" will do.

However wonderful and helpful it is to have a great teacher guide you, remember at all times that *you* are your own best teacher. Learn to trust your intuition again. Something that we've been conditioned to no longer do. Learn to back off when you need to. Learn to challenge yourself when you feel it in you.

You are powerful beyond measure, my dear.

"I am powerful beyond measure"

The End - Closing Your Practice

Each time you end your practice, notice the ease and energy you are feeling. Seal it all in to take out on a rainy day. It's nourishment for the soul. Take it into your day and the rest of your week and notice how you start navigating your life with more ease in your body and clarity in the mind.

Shavasana. Check-In.

Shavasana or "Corpse Pose" is the very last Yoga posture of the practice. It offers one last wonderful opportunity to check in with yourself. Lie on your back, your knees bent or extended, your arms by your side or on your belly, wherever comfortable. Put on any layers or cover up with a blanket if needed.

For a richer experience and to allow your body and mind to process the activity of your practice, don't ever skip this delicious step.

Check-in. Just as we did at the beginning. The most powerful indicator of change is your own awareness. Can you find a difference between before and after?

Take a few moments here to scan your body and mind. Then relax, and allow yourself to drop any muscular effort or focus. Stay awake. Give yourself permission to process everything. Stay with yourself for another few moments here.

You might drift in the expansive energy you feel in and around your body, a sense of transcendence even. If it's been a strong practice, you might doze off to the relaxing sounds of either your slow and gentle breathing or the sounds of the music your teacher might be playing. All is good.

You might find that once your mind no longer has a specific focus, it might start to get a little noisier again, ready to entertain with shopping lists or dinner or the week ahead. Turn away from the struggle of needing to "stop your thoughts".

Instead, gently move your focus to the subtle energy within: Notice any buzzing through the body, the temperature, your heartbeat, the pulse of life within you, and the spaciousness you created within.

Just for a little longer, enjoy the stillness & peace within you.

Gratitude

"It's the experience of counting one's blessings." And right after Relaxation, it is a powerful time and space to practice gratitude.

One amazing ability we have as humans is that we can actively choose what to focus on. When we feel centred, relaxed, and at ease, everything flows easily and it seems like we can handle everything that life throws at us.

So whatever your situation, you can decide to shift your focus to something positive. And gratitude is one of the best tools to do that.

"Gratitude is the feeling that embodies the word "Thank You". It is the unexpected reward of a kind deed that is magically produced by your brain. It is the cute, tingly feeling in your body that makes you smile at strangers." - The 5 Minute Journal

Gratitude rewires your brain to become happier and healthier. A regular practice of expressing and truly meaning it when you say the words Thank You has so many easily available benefits:

- It can make you more optimistic and positive about your life
- You need fewer visits to the doctor
- It can improve your sleep quality and reduce feelings of anxiety and depression
- Better moods and less fatigue
- Less inflammation, even reducing the risk of heart failure

Make it a habit to close your Yoga practice with three things you're grateful for right in the moment. Feeling gratitude takes your focus from a place of lack to one of abundance.

It could be anything – there is something wonderful to be found at all times.

Be grateful for the sunshine.
 Be grateful for your home.
 Be grateful for the delicious tea and nurturing food you eat.
 Be grateful for the stranger who shared a smile with you today.

Thank yourself for taking care of yourself.
 Thank your Higher Self (God, the Universe – whatever resonates) for supporting you, and for being there for you through the good and the

bad.

Say thank you to yourself for the last thing you accomplished today – even if that is simply doing the dishes or even just getting out of bed this morning.

Be grateful for your amazing, beautiful body for carrying you, for its fascinating mechanisms that work without us even being aware of it.

Be grateful for the light of a candle, for shining some light into the darkness and showing you the shadows but also the path ahead.

Beyond your practice, notice what happens when you tell your loved ones daily what you appreciate about them. It lightens up their days and that smile you receive in return will make you feel good too.

Journal it!

After every practice, write down what came up. Any changes physically. Thoughts. Mental activity. Emotions. Insights. Contemplations.

Writing down all of your personal thoughts and feelings can be very helpful in supporting emotional and mental health. It helps to clear your mind, reduce anxiety, gives you a break from obsessive thinking, and enables you to self regulate. It increases awareness and improves the perception of your practice and life, and even boosts physical health. The positive effects of journaling are even present when you don't get to write every day!

When you write down what's on your heart, you get it out of your system, and so you limit any strong influence these thoughts might have over you. You'll slowly start to better understand your needs, and as a result, you're better able to look after yourself and your well-being. You'll also stay on the path you're committed to and remind yourself why you're here on the mat in the first place.

There are many helpful journal invitations, prompts, and affirmations you can find. Here are a few of my regular go-to's to get you started:

- What thoughts came up during practice?
- What feelings were dominant?
- Did you react to any sensations, noises, or words by the teacher?
- What did the teacher say that stuck with you?
- How could today's practice have gone better?
- What was your intention for today's practice?
- What did you enjoy most about it?
- What progress did you see?
- What were your energy levels like today?
- Did you feel any niggles or pain?
- What are you most grateful for in terms of your practice today?
- What was your biggest challenge?

Use these prompts to get you started, though don't limit yourself to them. Use your journal as a record of your growth. For a sense of achievement, go back regularly to see how far you've come.

6

MONKEY MIND & MINDFUL MOMENTS

The mind is often compared to a monkey representing the qualities of being easily distracted, noisy, patronising, creating worst-case scenarios in downward spirals, and generally always on the go.

If you've ever been to a Buddhist temple, you might have seen a statue of an elephant and a monkey, both bowing to the Buddha, the "enlightened one". The monkey here characterises these more mind*less* qualities, whereas the elephant represents a calm and equanimous mind.

We have probably all experienced our very own monkey mind battling inside us before. That cheeky monkey taking the wheel trying to dominate what you think, do, and feel.

When you're starting a new habit of practicing Yoga, these battles are likely to happen as well. Of course they would, and you'll get very familiar with your monkey mind along the way:

"I can't do that" or
   "I'm not strong enough to do this"
   "I'm not flexible enough for this"
   "Not calm enough"
   "Haven't got my life together enough" ...

All these "not-being-enough's" are very restrictive, aren't they? Limiting and frustrating too if we keep entertaining them. It's not a happy place to be in.

Therefore, I challenge you to create a sense of acceptance around it. As you continue doing that, you're training your brain to find new connections, rewire your nervous system, find new growth opportunities, and move into the full capacity you have within your body. Give the monkey a banana and yourself permission to cut yourself some slack.

I invite you to create these small, but mindful moments:

- Whenever you notice your monkey mind creeping up - become aware of it! It sounds simple, but this "becoming aware of it" is hands down the biggest and often most difficult step to calm it.
- Notice which thoughts pop up. Notice the quality of them, what they are, and maybe even how they make you feel. Notice how repetitive they are. Notice what keeps coming back.
- Notice they're just that - thoughts and feelings. They come and go. The beauty is that we don't need to identify with them.
- Take a deep breath in - exhale completely.
- And then, draw your attention to your intention, to the reason why you're practicing, and gently move ahead with what you were doing before.

Then consciously draw your mind back into this present moment. Give 100% of your energy to your practice when you're on your mat. Or the person you're with or the task at hand - for a deeper connection and a richer quality of life.

By creating these small mindful moments on your Yoga mat, you are cultivating laser-beam-like focus and concentration. To more easily come back home to yourself, your centre. By re-framing the discomfort or the grateful pain as a good sign, the benefits that come with consistent practice will soon become apparent in your life.

When you go to your first class or join me online, you're given posture cues, breathing and movement cues as well as invitations to check in with yourself often. Continuously observe how you feel, where you feel sensations, and what thoughts arise. Or thinking patterns – what comes up a lot or which postures do you tend to resist or don't like at all? (It's said these are the ones we should focus on most!)

Know where you are right now. Though don't worry about where that is or what that looks like. Do not worry about how flexible or inflexible you are.

Instead, give yourself permission to enjoy moving, enjoy discovering a new relationship with your body. The fact you're on your mat practicing is a huge step. And hey, you've done that already, so give yourself a pat on the back.

And when negative or frustrating thoughts do show up – and they most likely will again and again – here's the trick again:

Catch them when they pop up. Step back.
Know they're just that: Thoughts.

Once you start doing this every time you practice, it will become a habit and you'll also find yourself noticing more subtle, beautiful situations in your life off the mat.

7

CREATING LASTING CHANGE

"Tapas" in Sanskrit means "heat" and can be translated as self-discipline, spiritual effort, and change. It's our determined effort to follow through and create transformation in our lives.

Start Your Transformation Today

Tapas, or Self-Discipline, is one of the Niyamas, which together with the Yamas are foundational to all Yogic thoughts.

It's the day-to-day choice to burn away non-supportive habits. Instead, we dedicate ourselves to choosing to move away from or give up instant pleasure for future rewards. We're playing the long-term game, becoming stronger in our bodies and minds.

We practice *tapas* by continuing to show up for ourselves for a regular practice ("Sadhana") and in the loving words of Deborah Adele: *"Like a drop of water eventually shapes a rock, the consistency of practice over time brings the change and fulfillment. We offer ourselves to the next higher version of us".*

Practical Tips to Create Change

To get started anywhere, we need to commit to creating space in our lives to establish a new, powerful routine that moves us toward our intention.

As we discussed earlier, create an environment that makes it as easy as possible to follow through and get set up:

- Remember your intention: what is your big why?
- Schedule it: same time, same day if possible
- Add a reminder to make it real!
- Make it non-negotiable: Never let it slide to the bottom of your list
- Journal it: a powerful tool for progress & celebrating results
- Be kind to yourself. Always.

We all know that change isn't easy. We resist it, it's scary and uncomfortable. You will come up to mental and physical obstacles along the way. The practice itself will challenge you as you step out of your comfort zone.

Though by doing the groundwork, you are more likely to remain clear and strong in your intention along the way, so that old habits and distractions will have less power over you, and slowly dissolve. And so that you can go on to enjoy cultivating strength and growth, freedom and ease within all areas of your life.

You are starting to create a beautiful flow of communication within your body and mind. On a cellular level, you are creating new neural pathways. And every time you dive in with more precision, you generate more strength and control. You start to hold yourself differently. You may even grow physically as you stand tall, feeling more confident in yourself. More grounded. And yes, coming from a stronger core within.

"Stick with it, follow through and never ever quit on yourself."- Marie Forleo

The journey is the real goal.

Allow yourself right now, to let go of having to know or be able to do everything straight away. Let go of the "end-gaming", the urge to get into the full Yoga posture right now, without your body willing or able to follow suit.

As you become familiar with that sweet point of awareness, realise the beautiful opportunity and powerful ability to switch thoughts around and shift things for you. To create change for the better.

"I am strong and trust my intuition"

8

JUST FOR YOU!

A free gift to you, wonderful reader.

YOGA
MOVEMENT &
MEDITATION

nourish body, mind & soul

To get you started with your practice on the mat, and as a thank you for reading my book, I would love to invite you to practice with me online! Go to:

https://evejuniper.com/practical-guide-book-thank-you

Get ready to play!

9

CONCLUSION

Really well done on getting started on your Yoga journey! To wrap up our time together, here are five key things to remember for your time ahead:

1. **Breathe.** Your breath is probably *the* single most important factor of the practice. Powerful beyond measure.
2. **Tune in.** Notice. Observe. Continuously. Without expectations or judgment. Deepen your awareness every time you step onto your mat.
3. **Set an intention.** Why do you want to practice? Cultivate and maintain focus. Allow it to act as a moving meditation on your mat.
4. **Challenge yourself to your edge.** Though never fight your bodies' clever mechanisms. Take your time.
5. Above all, **be mindful and be kind** to yourself. Cut yourself some slack as you embark on this powerful journey to reconnect to your gorgeous self.

I hope that you start recognizing a sense of your own beauty, your own powerful presence, knowing that you can live with more ease, feeling grounded and centred within. Allow your breath to continue to be your guiding light as you move through your practice, dedicated to move ahead, finding strength and lightness, love, and kindness for yourself.

And wherever you are on your journey through Perimenopause or Menopause, even when you feel you're *just* able to move your head (in pain), even when it takes you twenty minutes to get out of bed in the morning as every part of your body is in pain. Even when the option to go to a Yoga class is completely out of the question. If you continue connecting to your breath, in slow, conscious and mindful movements, with awareness to what is going on in and around you – you are practicing Yoga.

It is surrendering to each moment, being fully present with yourself. Drawing in your resources, to move inward and knowing that in fact you are *not* falling apart. You are simply on a journey of letting go of the old and welcoming the new.

Like a caterpillar, we're transitioning through Menopause. Leaving behind what no longer serves us. Don't hold onto it. Welcome the time to reflect and become more conscious and aware of your inner and outer world. When we tune in to work with ourselves, rather than fighting against, we can re-frame this time as an empowering chapter in our lives, one to fully embrace and be grateful for.

"A switch goes on that signals changes in our temporal lobes, a region in the brain that's associated with enhanced intuition." (Christiane Northrup).

Notice the shifts in the months and years to come. Enjoy the journey – now. Enjoy being curious, making this the start of an amazing relationship with yourself, re-connecting on a deeper level to shape and live your most amazing life.

However difficult it will often be, I hope that your practice leaves you feeling empowered, energised and nourished. And that then you realise that the only place you really need to look is inside you. Where all the answers for your deep inner questions lie. All will be revealed in due time. Including the bright light that I already know you have within. Let it shine.

Now just as I love closing my Yoga classes together with my students, I invite you to join me here:

Take your palms together in front of your heart. Bow your head to your fingertips, towards your beautiful self. Take a deep breath in. And exhale it all out.

Take a moment of gratitude toward yourself, your beautiful body, your practice, as well as the strength, the love and commitment within you to show up for yourself and everyone in your life.

"May you stay present to the sensations, and your reactions to those sensations, and be granted insight to perceive yourself more clearly without judgment, disappointment or shame. Let this practice release the tension effectively, unleashing any repressed emotions that are blocking you from your truest nature and most divine self.

Let this practice nourish you deeply and bring about healing.
May this practice be blessed. May there be peace."
– Seane Corn

And now - curl the ends of your mouth into a big smile.

Namaste
"The divine light within me
bows to the divine light
within you."

In gratitude to you, with much love and light,
Eve Juniper
Bristol, March 2023

10

REFERENCES & RESOURCES

Barry Popik, B. P. (2013, March 29). *"When the student is ready, the teacher will appear."* The Big Apple. Retrieved November 24, 2021, from http://web.archive.org/web/20200808144954/ht tps://www.barrypopik.com/index.php/new_york_city/entry/when_t he_student_is_ready_the_teacher_will_appear/

Corn, S. C. (n.d.). *Seane Corn, May we ask.* Sean Corn. Retrieved November 25, 2021, from https://seanecorn.com

Neurohealth Associates. (2020, July 4). *Neuroscience Reveals: Gratitude Literally Rewires Your Brain to be Happier.* NeuroHealth. Retrieved November 23, 2021, from https://nhahealth.com/neuroscience-rev eals-gratitude-literally-rewires-your-brain-to-be-happier/

A quote by Lao Tzu. (n.d.). https://www.goodreads.com/quotes/13395 72-when-the-student-is-ready-the-teacher-will-appear-when

Sutton, J., PhD. (2023, February 9). *5 Benefits of Journaling for Mental Health.* PositivePsychology.com. https://positivepsychology.com/bene

fits-of-journaling/

Intelligent Change. (n.d.). *The Five Minute Journal - Original Linen.* https://www.intelligentchange.com/products/the-five-minute-journal

Yoga Philosophy

Adele, D. (2009).*The Yamas & Niyamas: Exploring Yoga's Ethical Practice*(40081st ed.). On-Word Bound Books.

Gabriel, R. G. (2019, August 24).*Yoga Sutras 101: Everything You Need to Know.* Chopra. Retrieved November 24, 2021, from https://www.chopra.com/articles/yoga-sutras-101-everything-you-need-to-know

Yoga Sutras of Patanjali. (n.d.). Sutras.Yoga. Retrieved November 23, 2021, from https://sutras.yoga

What is the Meaning of Om? Discover the Origin of Om | Gaia. (n.d.). Gaia. https://www.gaia.com/article/what-meaning-om

Menopause & Hormones

Gottfried, S., & Northrup, C. (2014).*The Hormone Cure: Reclaim Balance, Sleep and Sex Drive; Lose Weight; Feel Focused, Vital, and Energized Naturally with the Gottfried Protocol*(Reprint ed.). Scribner.

Northrup, C. N. (2012).*The Wisdom of Menopause. Creating Physical and Emotional Health During the Change*(newly revised and updated ed.). Bantam Books.

Vitti, A. (2014).*WomanCode: Perfect Your Cycle, Amplify Your Fertility, Supercharge Your Sex Drive, and Become a Power Source*(Reprint ed.). HarperOne.

Practice with me online

Get ready to play! https://evejuniper.com/practical-guide-book-thank-you

Printed in Great Britain
by Amazon